Tight Hip Flexors

The Ultimate Guide to Curing Hip Flexor Pain

Table of Contents

Introduction

Over the course of our lives, it is likely that we will all experience varying episodes of pain in many joint locations. The most common areas of pain in the general population include: back, hip and knee. It may be difficult to determine the exact cause of pain without a thorough examination by a physician. However, many times pain can be significantly alleviated with exercise, stretching and improving postural attention. One common cause of discomfort is the *hip flexor* muscle group. Hip flexors are an essential muscle group that allows us to stand upright and to walk. This muscle group is used constantly throughout the day and is typically very strong. However, due to lifestyle and overuse, the hip flexors can become very tight and contribute to pain in the hip and the back. This book will review the functional anatomy of hip flexors, as well as their implication on mobility. In addition, you will learn how stretching your hip flexors can reduce pain and improve flexibility, with specific stretching guidelines. So, if you feel that you are limited by pain in your hips or back, consider the role of the hip flexors and begin a stretching routine today.

Hip Flexion

Hip flexion is term that is used in the medical field to specify a specific motion of the body. The hip joint is comprised of the top of the femur (long bone of the thigh) and the acetabulum (the "socket" of the pelvis). Flexion refers to a bending movement around a joint, which decreases the angle between the bones. A hip joint is straight when you are standing straight upright. When you flex your hip, your leg is elevated and the leg comes closer to your trunk. An easy way to refer to hip flexion is *bending your hip*.

In comparison, hip extension refers to joint movement in which you are increasing the angle between the bones. Hip extension is easily referred to as *straightening your hip*.

The hip flexors are responsible for these common movements:

- Bending your leg toward your body

- Bringing your trunk forward

- Pulling your knees upward

- Moving your legs from side to side and back to front

- Stabilizing your legs when standing on one leg

- Stabilizing your balance when standing

Anatomy Review

Muscle contraction elicits joint movement when it crosses a joint, which is really simple physics. Most muscles that create movement have an origin on one bone and an insertion point on another bone. The muscle belly typically crosses the joint. The joint is where two bones meet and where motion occurs. When the muscle concentrically contracts, the muscle shortens to pull one bone (where the muscle inserts) closer to the origin. Therefore, when the hip flexors contract, the leg is brought closer to the trunk.

The hip flexor group crosses the hip joint and pelvis, with some muscles originating in the back. The main bony structures that are involved in the hip flexor group include:

- **Vertebral column:** Your vertebral column is another term for your spine. Your spine begins at the base of your head and runs down your back to reach your pelvis. The lumbar spine and sacrum/coccyx are the areas of the spine that relate to your low back and tailbone.

- **Pelvis:** Your pelvis is made of the ilium and ischium, which are the top and bottom portions of the pelvis. The sacrum and coccyx at the base of the spine, meet in between the right and left sides of your pelvis.

- **Femur:** The femur is the long bone of your upper thigh. The femur joins the pelvis in order to form your hip joint.

The hip flexors are a group of muscles that cross the front of the hip joint. The major muscles of the hip flexor group are the iliacus, psoas, and tensor fasciae latae. In addition, the rectus femoris, sartorias, pectinus and piriformis assist in movement and stabilization.

Major hip flexor muscles:

- **Psoas/Iliacus (iliopsoas):** The psoas muscle runs from your lower spine to the inside of your femur, near the groin. The iliacus muscle is connected to a large portion of the psoas (which is why they are often referred to as the iliopsoas muscle). The iliopsoas is the dominant muscle that is used when lifting up your leg. It has the strongest pull and most compressing effect on the spine. The Iliopsoas is attached to the lumbar spine, so can create pain and compression at the spine if it is tight.

- **Tensor Fasciae Latae (TFL):** The TFL is located right at the top of your pelvis, more laterally. It then connects to form the iliotibial band (which runs down the side of the leg and inserts below the knee). The TFL is primarily used to stabilize the leg in episodes of single leg stance.

Supplemental hip flexor muscles:

- **Rectus Femoris:** The rectus femoris is part of the quadriceps muscle group. It crosses both the hip and the knee joints. The role of this muscle is to flex the hip and extend the knee.

- **Sartorius:** The Sartorius is important for leg movements that involve multiple planes. You use the Sartorius when you move your leg across your body and rotate your hip. Example: kicking a soccer ball or sitting with your leg crossed. The Sartorius is the longest muscle in the body.

- **Pectineus:** The pectineus is a small muscle that starts at the pubic region of the pelvis and connects on the inside of the femur. This muscle pulls the leg back and to the middle.

- **Piriformis:** The piriformis is a small, triangular muscle that inserts at the top of the femur and the base of the pelvis. The main purpose of the piriformis is to rotate your leg outward.

As you can see, the notion of a *tight hip flexor* is actually rather incorrect. It should actually be referred to as *tight hip flexors*! The action of these muscle groups together is what creates the bending movement of hip flexion.

What is a Tight Hip Flexor?

A tight hip flexor is a state in which one or more of the hip flexors lack full extension and flexibility. Tight hip flexor muscles are not able to fully straighten, but are limited in a shortened state. A tight hip flexor muscle belly is not supple, but instead is held in a tightened state. Sometimes, tight hip flexors feel tender to touch, with increased muscle tension. Tight hip flexors are caused by a variety of situations, lifestyle habits, and activity levels.

What Causes Tight Hip Flexors?

Typically, people develop tight hip flexors over time. Because hip flexor muscles cross in front of the hip joint, they are extended through walking. The very nature of standing and walking upright promotes appropriate hip flexor length. However, there are many situations in which you can develop tight hip flexors.

Prolonged sitting and sedentary lifestyles: In general, much of our population leads a sedentary and inactive lifestyle. Instead of engaging in physical activity and working outdoors, many people now sit on the couch, watching television or sitting on the internet. Many people spend far too much time sitting throughout their day, not allowing the hip flexors to stretch into extension.

Office jobs/prolonged computer work: As technology has increased, the physical activity of our work life has decreased. Many people spend most of their days seated at a desk with very little need to stand, walk and physically exert themselves. Sitting for most of the day puts the hip flexors in a shortened state (think: when sitting your hips are flexed with the legs in a position up near your trunk). It is no wonder that some of us feel stiff when arising to stand from our desks after a full day at the office. Unless people actively work to keep appropriate muscle length, it is likely that the cycle of prolonged desk work will continue to reinforce tight hip flexors.

Athletics/running: Just as sedentary individuals are prone to tight hip flexors, so too are athletes. For athletes that focus on running sports or distance running, the hip flexor muscle group can become overdeveloped and lack proper flexibility.

If athletes do not focus on stretching, they can easily acquire shortened hip flexor muscles overtime.

Poor posture: Many individuals with poor posture hold their pelvis in a position of anterior pelvic tilt. The abdominal muscle are weak, the pelvis is forward and there is excess curvature in the low back. This position of poor posture is associated with tight hip flexors and further promotes tightening of the hip flexors.

Tight Hip Flexors and Hip Pain

Anterior (front) hip pain: Snapping hip pain occurs when a muscle (or tendon, ligament) rolls over a bony prominence around the hip. When this happens at the front of the hip, it usually involves the iliopsoas muscle and tendon. This is common in runners and athletes. In this situation, the hip muscles are used excessively and become tired, tight and even inflamed.

Lateral (side) hip pain: Snapping hip pain can also occur over the side of the hip. When this happens at the side of the hip, it is related to tightness in the iliotibial band. The ITB rolls over the side of the femur and can cause discomfort and audible snapping sound.

Groin pain: Individuals experience groin pain when there is strain to the muscles of the inner thigh, such as the gracilis, pectineus, or adductor brevis/longus. These muscles contribute to inner thigh stability and can be easily strained when performing athletic activity, or when horseback riding or excessive stretching. In addition, tightness in these muscle groups can limit range of motion and contribute to stiffness in the hip joint.

Excess strain on this muscle group during activities that involve sprinting and kicking. Runners are more prone to hip flexor injuries due to repetitive overuse during the action of running. Slipping and falling can cause hip flexor issues. When the muscles are suddenly stretched beyond their normal capacity, you can experience hip and groin pain. For non-athletes, tightness in the hip flexors creates pain the hips that is experienced as stiffness. The stiffness is usually a dull, ache.

It is typically felt when first standing up from sitting or beginning to walk.

Tight Hip Flexors and Back Pain

Tightness in the hip flexors creates an anterior pelvic tilt. The pelvis has a lot of mobility and it can move forward (anterior) and backward (posterior). With an anterior pelvic tilt, your buttocks sticks out more than it should and your pelvis points forward/downward. Too much anterior tilt is bad for your posture and is known to contribute to low back pain. When your pelvis points forward/downward, your hamstrings (muscles in the back of your thighs) will become overstretched and work less efficiently. You will have excessive lumbar lordosis, meaning there will be an excessive amount of forward curve in your low back. Unfortunately this can be very harmful to the intervertebral discs, especially for the low lumbar spine.

This can impact the alignment of the entire spinal column and cause a forward head posture and even pain in the upper back, between the shoulder blades. In this position, the abdominals are usually weak, and the stomach is pushed forward. Weak abdominal muscles and weak back extensor muscles also contribute to this pattern of low back pain. Without adequate length in the iliopsoas muscle group, you cannot stand tall and overtime, it can lead to a hunched back posture. In addition, you will lack appropriate movement in your hips.

Improving your flexibility in the hip flexors can correct anterior pelvic tilt, especially when you also include strengthening exercises for your core muscles and buttocks muscle groups. To maintain the proper curvature of the spine, the muscles that are located in the front and back of the hip and pelvis must function in balance and coordination. The proper muscle length and strength of these muscles will keep the pelvis in a neutral tilt and proper alignment. A neutral pelvic tilt is important to maintain proper distribution of pressure through the intervertebral discs. Proper pelvic alignment protects back health and aids in maintaining a tall, upright posture.

Why is Stretching Important?

As a kid and teenager, it seemed as though flexibility was a given. With age it seems as though flexibility is more elusive and something that must be consciously improved. Lifestyle habits and muscle weakness contribute to poor muscle function. In addition, running sports creates muscle shortening. Therefore, we must make a conscious effort to work on our flexibility in order to improve our mobility and decrease aches and pains.

How to Stretch

When muscles are tight, they limit the range of motion of the joints that they cross. This limited range of motion can lead to improper joint mechanics while walking or performing daily tasks, in addition to poor posture. Follow these strategies to improve your flexibility:

- **Assess your flexibility**. Are you flexible? Are you tight? Do you have any idea? Take a couple of minutes and assess your own flexibility to determine your baseline starting point. Some people are naturally more flexible than others and women are typically more flexible than men. To test your hip flexor muscle flexibility, lay on your stomach with your legs extended. Then bend your knee to bring your heel toward your buttocks. Do you feel a stretching in the front of your thigh and hip?

  While you are assessing your flexibility, check other body parts. Try to sit with your legs extended in front of you. Can you reach down and touch your toes? This is a test for hamstring flexibility in the back of your legs. For your upper body, try to make your opposite hands touch behind your back, near your shoulder blades. This is a great indication of upper body flexibility. Also, you can assess any areas that you are having discomfort. More than likely, in the area of discomfort, you will have associated muscle tightness.

- **Static Stretching**. This may be the simplest form of improving flexibility, but it is effective. Stretching is accomplished when you place the muscle in an extended position to stretch the muscle fibers. For example, the role of the hip flexor muscle is to bend the hip. So, in order to stretch the hip flexor muscle group, you must fully extend the hip and straighten the trunk.

Static stretching should place the muscle in an elongated position for an extended period of time. Research shows that it takes 20-30 seconds to make a change in the length of the muscle fibers during static stretching. Therefore, aim to hold static stretches for 30 seconds and repeat several times.

Typically if you bring a joint to the fullest position of bending or straightening, you will be able to achieve a good stretch. Stretching should always be comfortable and should be done in a slow and sustained manner. Never bounce or push into pain when stretching.

- **Yoga**. Yoga is an age old form of exercise that teaches mind and body control for mental and physical health. There are various forms of yoga, all with benefits of improving flexibility. Hatha yoga is a traditional form of yoga that incorporates series of movements in slow, controlled and purposeful manner. Power yoga is essentially yoga with brawn. It incorporates continuous movements, creating an intense muscle building and cardiovascular workout. Hot yoga is a current craze which incorporates traditional yoga movements in a hot climate of 105 degree rooms. This hot climate promotes increased muscle flexibility and perspiration. Whatever style you decide to try, all yoga will promote whole body flexibility and body resistance strengthening. Try finding a class at your local health club, park district or even a yoga exercise video.

- **Pilates**. Pilates is a form of exercise that incorporates mind and body. Pilates promotes long, lean muscles, a clear mind and a refreshed sense of accomplishment. The exercises combine elements from yoga, breathing techniques, dancing, gymnastics and boxing. Joseph Pilates founded the principles of Pilates over 80 years ago. Basic Pilates exercises do not require any fitness equipment. Many exercises can be done on the floor, using your own body weight for resistance. More advanced exercisers may perform Pilates movements on exercise equipment called reformers.

- **Dance**. Dance is a wonderful form of exercise because it allows you to move your body in a rhythmic manner through a variety of positions. People who regularly danced throughout their lives are known to have better balance and less joint issues as compared to non-dancers. Dance is known to improve muscle strength and flexibility, while burning serious calories. Specifically, ballet and ballroom dancing are excellent forms for increasing flexibility.

- **Tai Chi**. Tai Chi is an ancient balance/flexibility/dance form of exercise that is shown to reduce stress and increase flexibility. The repetitive, deliberate and slow movements stretch the limbs through their full range of motion, stretching the muscles and maintaining good joint mobility. Tai chi is an excellent alternative to yoga for those who like exercise that combines mind and body.

Whatever form of flexibility exercise you engage in, make sure that you listen to your body and never stretch to the point of feeling pain. All stretches should feel comfortable yet challenging. You will find that with greater flexibility, you will have less pain, better muscle tone, and improved energy.

Specific Static Hip Flexor Stretches

In order to specifically improve the flexibility of the hip flexor muscle group, try incorporating some or all of these stretches into your workout routine. You will find that will improved flexibility in the hip flexor muscle group, you will be able to stand taller and move more freely in all of your activities.

When performing static stretches, try holding each position for 30 seconds. Aim to perform the 30 second stretch 2-5 times on each side. Use a watch with a second hand to ensure that you are actually holding the stretch for the entire duration. Many times, people quickly count or estimate 30 seconds, which ends up being much less. Alternate right and left legs in order to ensure equal stretching of both sides. It is not uncommon that you may find one leg to be more or less flexible than the other leg. Oftentimes this is due to physical activity and lifestyle habits. For example, a soccer player may have less flexibility in her dominant kicking leg in comparison to the other leg.

Remember that the stretches should never be painful. You should feel a moderate stretch that is comfortable and tolerable. Do not bounce in your stretch, but instead, allow your muscles to relax and elongate in a sustained hold.

Hip flexor stretch over stair: Place your foot on a step with your back leg firmly planted on the floor. Lean forward until you feel a stretch across the front of your hip. Depending on how far you stretch, you will feel a stronger or lighter stretch. Repeat on both legs.

Video: https://www.youtube.com/watch?v=8z_lO5hcCvU

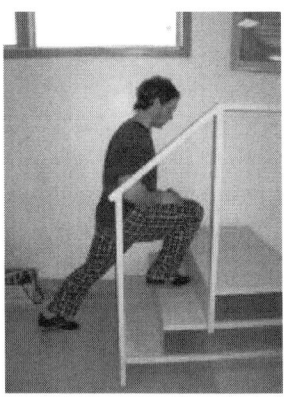

Standing hip flexor stretch (Yoga Warrior One): Step forward into a deep lunge position. Bring your arms overhead and lean your trunk backwards. Hold this position for a deep and comfortable stretch. Repeat with both legs by stepping forward with the opposite leg.

Video: https://www.youtube.com/watch?v=5rT--p_cLOc

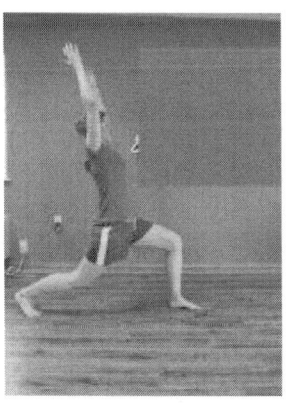

Half kneel stretch: Start by kneeling on the floor and then placing one foot up on the floor (half kneeling position). Next, lean forward with your trunk and allow your front knee to bend. You will feel a stretch along the front of the opposite hip. Hold this position for a comfortable stretch. Remember to keep your trunk upright and standing tall.

Video: https://www.youtube.com/watch?v=YQmpO9VT2X4

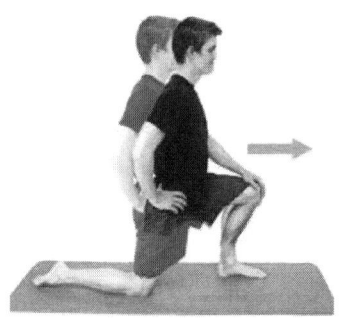

Standing Quadriceps Stretch: Stand in front of a chair, holding the back of the chair with one hand for balance. Bend your knee and bring your heel up toward your buttocks, holding with the hand on the same side of the body. Keep your back still and your chest upright. Avoid bending forward with your trunk. Pull until you feel a stretch in the front of your thigh. Repeat for both legs.

Video: https://www.youtube.com/watch?v=1Pik2RuIQZk

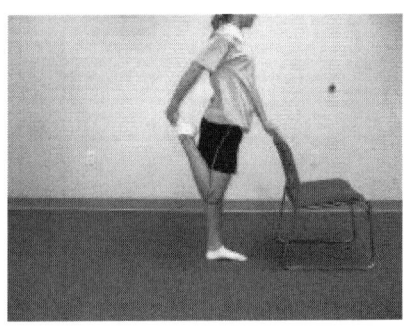

Iliopsoas Stretch over Chair: Place one knee on a chair. Your other leg should be in front of the chair. Keep your core muscles engaged, by tightening your abdominals to keep your back straight. Gently and slowly bend the front knee and move the body forward until you feel a stretch in the front of your opposite hip. The leg that is over the chair is the one being stretched. Repeat for both legs.

Video: https://www.youtube.com/watch?v=wUj8DXlGoCg

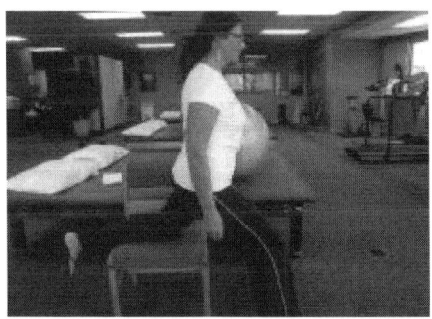

TFL (Tensor Fasciae Latae) Stretch: Sit on the floor with legs extended. Cross one leg over the other and pull the knee toward your chest. Pull until you feel a stretch in the side of your hip. Repeat for both legs.

Video: https://www.youtube.com/watch?v=SlvgfhQKIEA

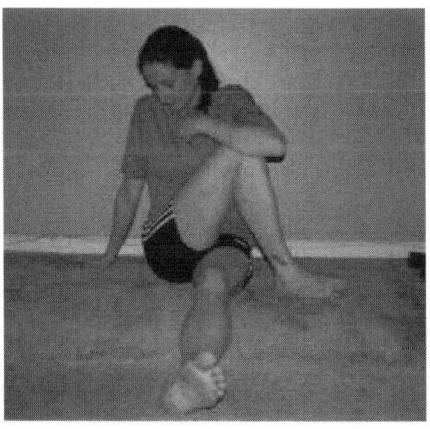

Supine knee to chest: Lie on a high bed or mat table, toward the edge. Let your leg hang off the edge of the bed and lower toward the floor until you feel a stretch along the front of your thigh. Then, bring the opposite knee up toward your chest for a deeper stretch. Do not allow your back to arch.

Video: https://www.youtube.com/watch?v=sQXilXUll-M

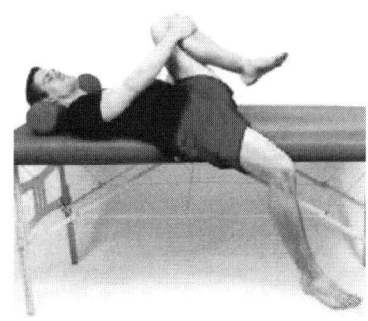

Heel to buttocks stretch: Lie on your stomach with both legs extended. Next, place a belt (or towel) around one lower leg. Pull the belt to bend your knee and pull your heel up toward your buttocks. Do not allow your pelvis to rise up; it should stay in contact with the floor. You should feel a stretch along the front of your hip and thigh. Repeat on the other leg.

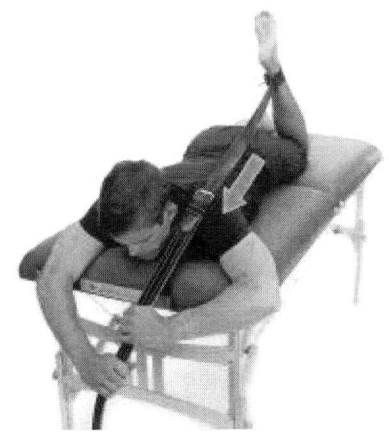

Butterfly Stretch: Lie on your back with your knees bent. Place the bottom of your feet together and lower your knees to each side. You should feel a stretch on your inner thighs. Allow your muscle to relax and feel a deep, but comfortable stretch.

Video: https://www.youtube.com/watch?v=rdxD3POKbV8

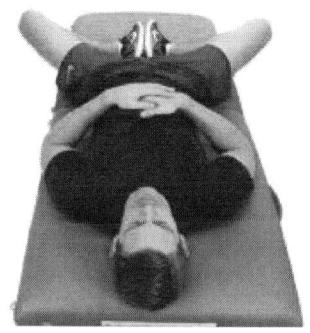

Adductor (inner thigh) Stretch: Lie on the floor with your hips as close to the wall as you can get them. Your legs should be straight and resting against the wall. Allow your legs to slide away from each other as gravity assists to stretch the inside of your thighs.

Video: https://www.youtube.com/watch?v=3AhWDGojxJk

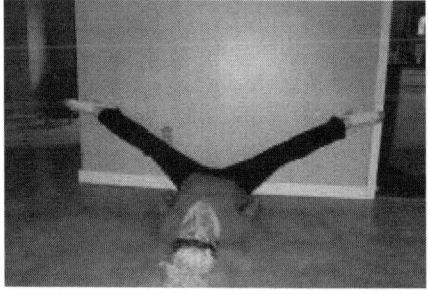

Pigeon Stretch: Place your bent leg in front of your body, with your other leg extended behind your body. Try to keep your pelvis pointing forward and then allow your trunk to lower toward the ground. Try to stay relaxed and do not move into a painful position. Repeat this stretch for the other leg.

Video: https://www.youtube.com/watch?v=FVlX5HNKamw

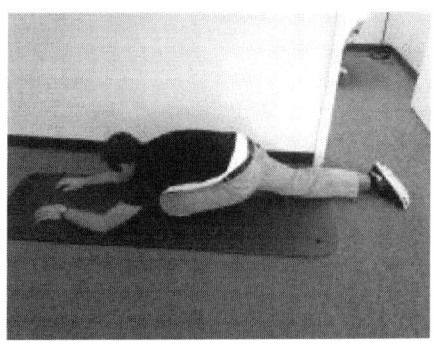

Cobra: Lie on your stomach with your arms placed under your shoulders. Keep your palms flat and press up, extending your trunk. To increase the stretch across your hips, lift your upper body until a stretch is felt. This will also improve your back strength.

Video: https://www.youtube.com/watch?v=JDcdhTuycOI

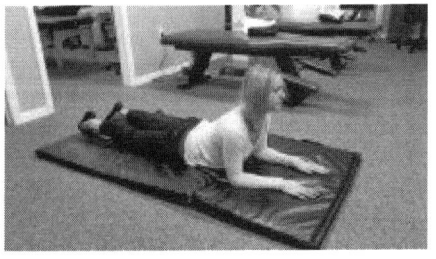

Postural Implications

In order to combat back pain that is associated with tight hip flexors, you must improve flexibility but also improve the strength of the back muscles. Improving back strength with improve posture and back health. A tall posture exudes confidence, class, health, and strength. Having good posture is something that takes some attention and practice. By working on your posture, you will increase your self-confidence. In addition, you will improve other aspects of your health. Good posture prevents negative effects on your physique. Some implications of poor posture include: increased belly fat, varicose veins, osteoporosis, weakening of the vertebral column, pinched nerves and back pain. That is plenty of reason to keep yourself standing tall. There are exercises you can do to improve your posture and keep good back strength.

Try these back strengthening exercises in combination with your flexibility training:

Rows: Stand up tall and with your arms at your side. Bend your elbows to 90 degrees, fists pointing forward. Row your arms back, like you are trying to pinch your shoulder blades together. You will be activating your postural control muscles in your upper back. Complete 15 repetitions and then perform three sets.

Pelvic tilts: Lay on your back with your knees bent and feet on the floor. Press your back into the floor by rolling your pelvis backwards. Then, roll your pelvis forward so your back arches away from the floor. Repeat this 15 times.

Bridges: Lay on your back with your knees bent and feet on the floor. Tighten your buttocks and abdominal muscles to lift your buttocks off the floor, creating a "bridge." Hold this bridge for 5 seconds and then slowly lower to the floor. Repeat this 15 times.

Sit on a ball: If you sit most of your day, like at a desk job, try switching out your chair for an exercise ball. By sitting on an exercise ball, you will have to engage your postural control muscles to keep your back straight.

Practice and attention: It is easy to fall forward into a slouched posture, especially while seated at work. Make an effort to pay attention to your posture and correct yourself when you find you are slouching. Over time, your good posture will become a habit and your norm.

Beginning to Exercise: Pain Vs. Soreness

So, what is wrong with pain? Pain is your body's signal to slow down or stop doing an activity. Pain is a sensory awareness of injury or dysfunction. Think about when you touch something hot. Your body immediately lifts your hand before you can even consciously detect how painful it is. This phenomenon is due to the withdrawal reflex, which is a spinal reflex that serves the purpose to protect the body from harm. Although the pain of an injury is not as immediate as the withdrawal reflex, it is still your body's way of telling you something is wrong. True pain that may be experienced during exercise would be described as: sharp, stabbing, or intense. Injuries can occur when beginning an exercise program and not using proper mechanics. If you begin to feel pain, you should stop what you are doing; adjust your intensity, position or activity. If the pain does not subside, seek guidance from a trusted professional.

On the other hand, muscle soreness is completely normal and expected. When exercising, your muscle builds new fibers and strength by undergoing tiny micro-tears. These small tears stimulate new muscle fiber repair and growth, which leads to increased muscle mass and strength. The phenomenon called delayed onset muscle soreness (DOMS) causes a feeling of muscle soreness typically 24-48 hours after exercise. This discomfort is typically described as soreness, achiness, or tightness. This discomfort is not associated with true injury, but instead a normal response to taxing a muscle. This soreness is normal and typically resolves within one or two days.

It is important to drink plenty of water to stay hydrated, which will decrease muscle soreness. When you are exercising, you need to pay attention to what your body is telling you. You should feel that your body is being challenged but you should not push into true pain. Determine if you are experiencing pain vs. soreness to ensure safe, injury free exercise.

Beginning to Exercise: Commitment

After reaching this, hopefully you have made a decision to improve the flexibility of your hip flexors (and other muscle groups)! It is important that you believe in your goals and make time for yourself to stretch and exercise. Leave no room for excuses: It will be easy to start making excuses for not exercising (did you really need to scrub your bathroom floor instead of going to yoga class?). Don't allow yourself to give into excuses. Keep yourself accountable for your fitness plan.

Make a plan and stick to it. Plan out your fitness schedule one week ahead of time. This way, you will have a plan going into each day as to what you will be doing for exercise. This will leave little room to accidentally run out of time in your day. You should look at stretching and exercise as an appointment with yourself. You would not cancel an appointment with a friend, so why should you cancel an appointment with yourself?

Set fitness goals. In your first week, start with small, obtainable goals. Make a goal to stretch for 15 minutes, on 3 days of the week. You can find 45 minutes in your entire week to work on your flexibility and improve your overall health. By reaching small fitness goals, you will be motivated to continue and even challenge yourself further the next week.

Avoid overtraining. Overtraining injuries result when you push your body too hard or too fast. Overtraining injuries can happen to athletes and amateurs and present in varying forms. Oftentimes, overtraining injuries present as pain, fatigue, decreased appetite, stiffness or decline in physical performance. To avoid overtraining injuries, it is important to realize that training and fitness goals need to be reasonable and appropriate for your fitness level. It is not smart to decide that you are going to run a marathon next week, when you have little experience or training in distance running. It is important to begin slowly and build up slowly.

In addition, it is important to fuel your body with nutritious food that provides good protein and healthy carbohydrates. You need to remember to drink adequate amounts of water and get plenty of rest. Exercise should begin with an appropriate warm up and finish with a slow cool down and stretching.

Conclusion

Improving the flexibility of your hip flexors is a great first step in protecting yourself from hip and back pain. Your increased flexibility will allow for greater ease in movement and improved ability to stand upright. Remember to avoid prolonged periods of sitting, which contributes to muscle shortening. Try to get up every hour while you are working and allow yourself to stand up straight and walk around. Practice good posture and keep yourself from developing a forward flexed position. After you feel confident in taking care of your hip flexors, consider other muscle groups. Do you have appropriate hamstring flexibility, back strength and Achilles length? Imagine if you had great flexibility throughout your body? How wonderful might you feel? Commit to stretching and flexibility exercises and you won't wake up feeling stiff!

20564334R00022

Printed in Great Britain
by Amazon